Grandma's Herbal Lore

Ancient Herbal Recipes and Remedies Volume 5

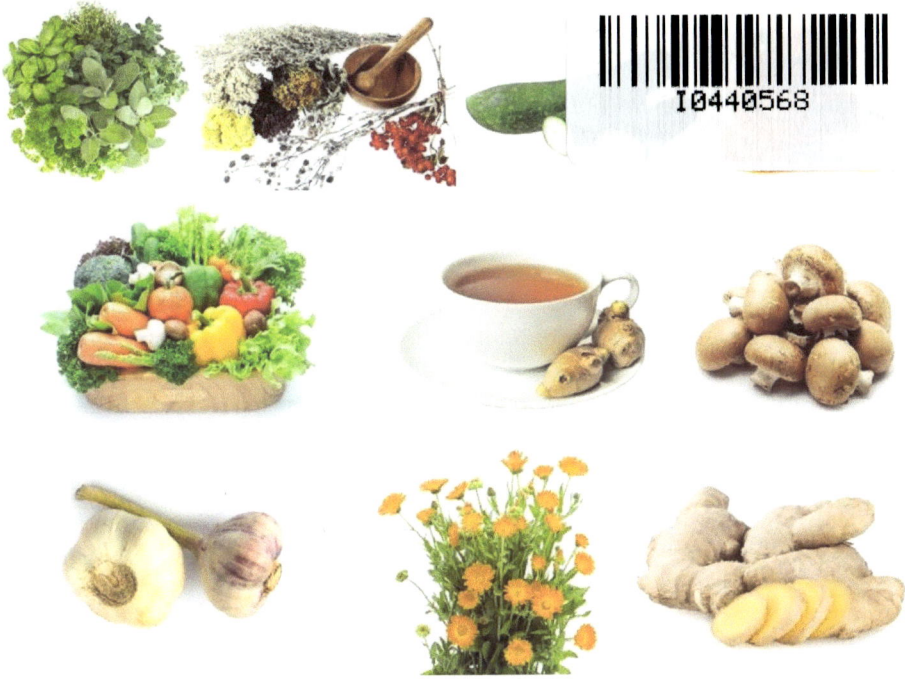

I0440568

Dueep Jyot Singh

Natural Remedy Series
Mendon Cottage Books

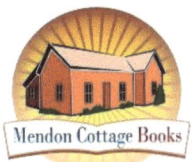

JD-Biz Publishing

Download Free Books!

http://MendonCottageBooks.com

Disclaimer

The information is this book is provided for informational purposes only. It is not intended to be used and medical advice or a substitute for proper medical treatment by a qualified health care provider. The information is believed to be accurate as presented based on research by the author.

The contents have not been evaluated by the U.S. Food and Drug Administration or any other Government or Health Organization and the contents in this book are not to be used to treat cure or prevent disease.

The author or publisher is not responsible for the use or safety of any diet, procedure or treatment mentioned in this book. The author or publisher is not responsible for errors or omissions that may exist.

Warning

The Book is for informational purposes only and before taking on any diet, treatment or medical procedure, it is recommended to consult with your primary health care provider.

Our books are available at

1. Amazon.com
2. Barnes and Noble
3. Itunes
4. Kobo
5. Smashwords
6. Google Play Books

Download Free Books!

http://MendonCottageBooks.com

Table of Contents

Introduction

In volume 5 of Grandma's natural remedies, with herbal lore and ancient recipes, you are going to get an excellent critique mixture of the knowledge of the ages, brought around to us through papyri , books and trial and error experiments done by the ancients. The word of mouth results, have been the product of years of experimentation done millenniums ago.

When did grandma become the epitome of wisdom and experience? Well, we should go back millenniums, when it was the job of the oldest generation to take care of the youngest generation, while the adults generation in between went out to collect food, water and other basic necessities necessary for survival.

The job of raising and training the children was left to those people who were most experienced. It is possibly this reason why the oldest and the youngest generations still find that they are more compatible and comfortable with each other, due to natural preference, instinctive selection and human psychological and social behavior.

So the children of the tribe, group, gathering, and city were put in charge of the elders, who used to talk to them about their ancient traditions, talk to them by their own grandparents. The rules and regulations of living in society and getting to know one's own place in the hierarchy of a tribe was thus transmitted from generation to generation through these elders.

Grandpa trained the kids with tribal knowledge and physical exercise. Grandma was in charge of their overall emotional, spiritual and physical well-being. She was responsible for their health, well-being, food and other essential things necessary to keep children healthy and well-balanced members of the family and later on the tribe.

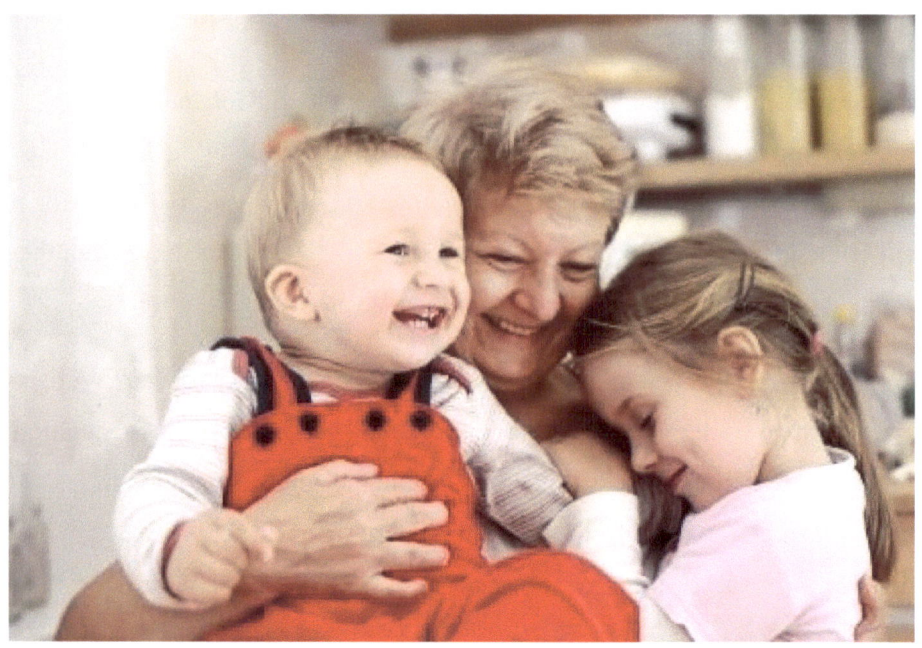

…and that caring instinct still is present…

That is why the matriarch – mother – was given the job of passing on the herbal knowledge to the girls in the family, preparing them to be future matriarchs taking care of their own families, as years went by. The boys were trained into becoming warriors, teachers, farmers, food gatherers or in other professions by the males of the tribe.

So the lines were demarcated out very clearly in well-regulated times since ancient days. The house, home and hearth and other duties pertaining to a domestic nature was under the jurisdiction of the females. The land, the preservation, cultivation and protection of the area around it was under the jurisdiction of the males.

So it was the man's prerogative to be the hunter and the warrior, to feed and protect his family and tribe.

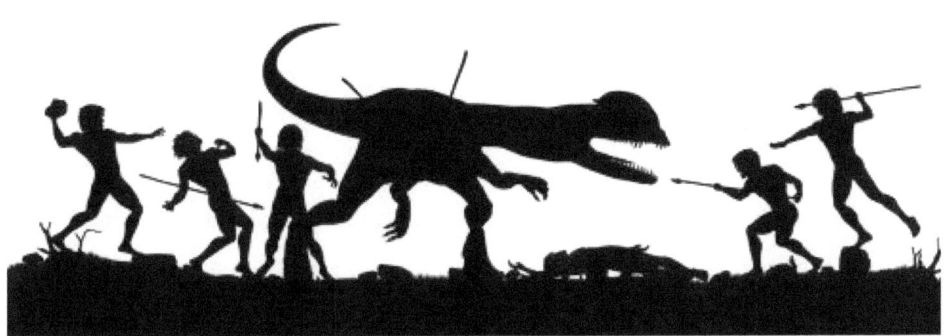

and so it has been down the ages...

 It was the woman's prerogative to take care of the well-being of the family by giving them proper meals and medicines when necessary.

This is the way animal tribes followed the hierarchy through millenniums. Naturally, man also had to follow the same rules and regulations. There was one leader, who used to take care of his tribe. The rest of the members of the tribe followed the rules set out by the tribe under pain of death for rebellion. This has been the natural law of every living species, since it appeared on the face of the earth.

That is why animal observers say that a young wolf is put immediately to death if it raises its eyes to an older wolf, and tries to take the elder's position in the hierarchy of the tribe. It is the job of mother and father Wolf to teach their cups how to behave. After they have been trained, their training is going to be done by the rest of the wolves in the pack.

Apply the same analogy to man through the centuries. Man, of course, did not kill his cubs when they showed rebelliousness, but he punished them, and taught them how to behave. Nevertheless, in Roman times, more than 3000 years ago a father had power of life and death over his children. Because at that time, it was still survival of the fittest.Man being a little more civilized and evolved began to set out rules for the training of the young wolves in his pack, by leaving everything to the elders. That is why the grandpas and the grandmas of the pack trained, taught and educated the children so that they could become useful members of the pack when they grew up to be adults.

Anyway, here is an enjoyable paragraph which was written by Kipling in Puck of Pook's Hill where a young Roman soldier describes his family life more than 2500 years ago.

"…But what lessons did you do - when - when you were little?' 'Ancient history, the Classics, arithmetic and so on,'he answered. 'My sister and I were thickheads, but my two brothers (I'm the middle one) liked those things, and, of course, Mother was clever enough for any six. She was nearly as tall as I am, and she looked like the new statue on the Western Road - the Demeter of the Baskets, you know. And funny! Roma Dea! How Mother could make us laugh!'

'What at?'

'Little jokes and sayings that every family has. Don't you know?'

'I know we have, but I didn't know other people had them too,' said Una.
'Tell me about all your family, please.'

'Good families are very much alike. Mother would sit spinning of evenings
while Aglaia read in her corner, and Father did accounts, and we four
romped about the passages. When our noise grew too loud the Pater would
say, "Less tumult! Less tumult! Have you never heard of a Father's right
over his children? He can slay them, my loves - slay them dead, and the
Gods highly approve of the action!" Then Mother would prim up her dear
mouth over the wheel and answer: "H'm! I'm afraid there can't be much of
the Roman Father about you!" Then the Pater would roll up his accounts,
and say, "I'll show you!" and then - then, he'd be worse than any of us!'

'Fathers can - if they like,' said Una, her eyes dancing.'Didn't I say all good
families are very much the same?'

So now you know the reason why grandma's natural remedies and ancient
recipes were considered to be effective, because she could not afford to have
the tribe and families thinned out due to disease and neglect, let us look at
what she has in store for us in volume 5.

Delicious, Refreshing Traditional Healthy Drinks

How to make the perfect Nimbu pani – lime juice

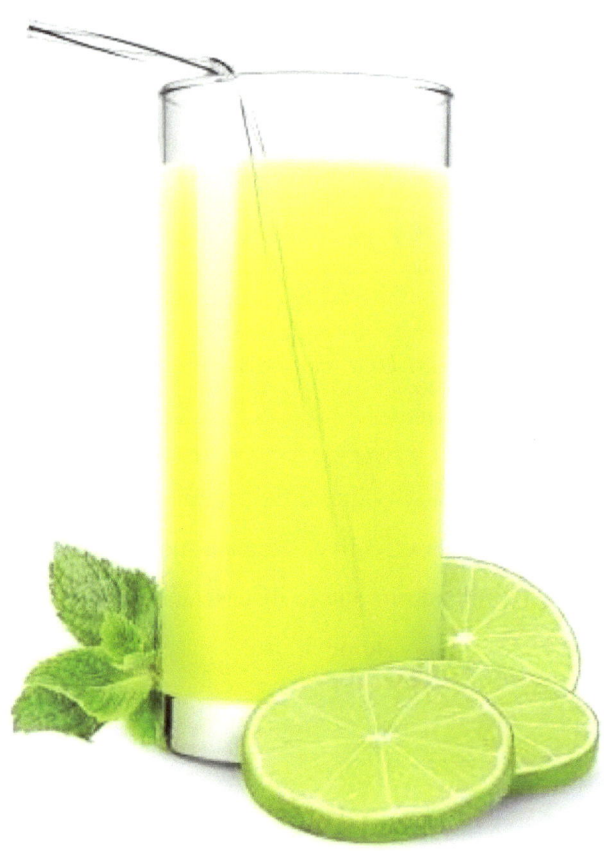

This particularly delicious drink is drunk in copious quantities all over the East, all throughout the summer. This can either be made at home, or you can buy it from any market lemon juice vendor. He is going to squeeze it right in front of you, and then top it up with soda, rocksalt, powdered cumin seed, lemon and pepper.

8 tsp. of honey, 6 tbsp. squeezed lime juice, 4 cups of water , salt to taste , crushed ice to serve. Mix them all together and place them in the fridge. Keep drinking whenever you want to replenish your vitamins C, energy, and water level. We kids managed about four-- 5 glasses of nimbu pani a day and never ever caught a cold in the winters or a sunstroke in the summers.

This nimbupani was also a blessing during the rare occasions when we caught a fever, because warm nimbu pani with lots of salt and pepper four times a day brought us bouncing back and in fighting trim within the week.

Apart from that, we had glowing complexions, because we did not mind rubbing the lime skins upon our cheeks to try to get rid of the sunburn! We have this habit of rubbing the skins of every single raw fruit we ate upon our faces and hands to see its effect. I must admit that apart from cooling us down and cleaning our epidermis, these fruit skins made sure that we never suffered from wrinkles or pimples.

Buttermilk

Another very healthy and refreshing drink of North India is called *Lassi.* (buttermilk.) Apart from its therapeutic uses, which I am going to list soon, it is the most refreshing drink anybody could ever have thought of.

One of my happiest memories as a child was coming down to the plains to our ancestral home, where we had an otherwise busy, busy, busy Dad all to ourselves. Being in holiday mode, he would spend his time, teaching us riding, shooting, fishing, swimming, and indulging in other hard physical survival, outdoor exercises and activities, which we could not do in our normal abodes – the mountains or the forests.

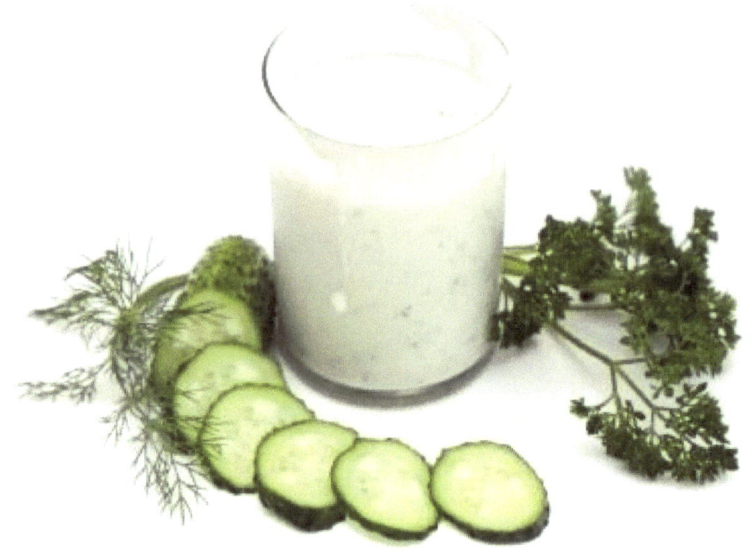

The middle eastern equivalent is salty yoghurt-Kefir.

Coming back after a hard morning's ride or swim, my grandmother would greet us with Lassi before we filled ourselves to the brim with traditional North Indian fare made in desi ghee with dollops of salted homemade butter swimming upon every imaginable surface.

- **Lassi:**

❖ **2 cups rich creamy yogurt.**

❖ **Equal amount of crushed ice or iced water.**

❖ **Two table spoons honey**

❖ **Pepper and salt to taste.**

❖ **A little powdered roasted cumin seeds for taste.**

In ancient times, when there were no mixers and grinders around, all these items were placed in a huge churn and churned by hand until the mixture was frothy. The butter, which came up to the surface was then gathered and fed to the family or sold in the city, every day. 3000 years ago, the society of the East was agriculture-based and as it is still done in Africa, the richness and prosperity of a tribe or its people was based on the number of cows it had.

This buttermilk was topped off with a slice of cream or yogurt and fed to anybody coming into the house, after a hard days work. It was also the usual accompaniment to every meal. This should clearly indicate that the ancients were not bothered about dieting. In fact the Oriental equivalent of beauty is 44 – 36 – 44. And that can only be obtained on a steady diet of Lassi , cream, butter and other milk-based delicious goodies, which make life so worth living.

Buttermilk As a Cancer Cure

Lassi is known as the food of the gods and in ancient Ayurveda treatises , it was supposed to heal many ills. In fact, cancer has supposedly been cured by feeding the patient a steady diet of *just grapes* (nothing else at all) for a month and then adding lassi to the diet until he is cured completely.

I really do not know whether this has been proved, because the idea of cancer was not a part of Eastern medicine until the 17th century when it was brought to the notice of the Orientals from their Western medical counterparts. No doubt we had some concept of odd outgrowths and tumours and these were cured by grapes and *lassi. But they were not treated under the term "cancer."*

However, I am not looking at the idea of **curing cancer** with a steady diet of fruit and vegetables, as something quite impossible.

Because the proof of the pudding is right in my family, my mother's cousin, who was suffering from cancer, is now completely cured. But she only eats raw fruit, raw vegetables and drinks only fresh fruit juices. She has stopped eating cooked food. And she is still going strong, 30 years after doctors gave up on her, and after being clinically declared dead twice! So, I believe that this natural diet is powerful enough to cure you, even in the most drastic of circumstances and cases and best of luck. You may want to try and test out this cure, along with a fruit and vegetable diet. Again, God go with you.

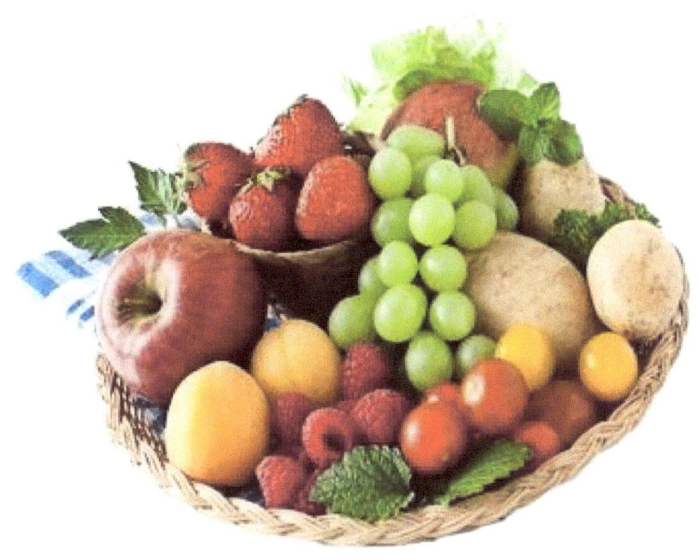

Fresh fruit and herbs and their juices? Excellent.

For Victims Of Strokes

A stroke can happen to anyone.

It is rather terrible to have a member of your family struck down by paralysis or a stroke. In villages, many of the cases were rather miraculously cured by feeding the patients regularly with fresh meat of wood pigeons, as soon as the stroke victim is hit.

Apart from this, a regular diet of hoof soup (hooves of oxen or sheep are best) would have the patient on his feet again, God willing. This diet has to be interspersed with a regular massage of warm mustard oil upon the affected areas.

- One of the well-known remedies is grinding five cloves of garlic with 10 g of honey. This mixture is spread upon whole-wheat tacos (*rotis*) and fed to the patient twice a day.

- Add five cloves of garlic to 10 g of sesame oil, and bring the mixture to a boil. Feed the patient this either spread upon a Taco or raw, if he can manage to drink it. This is going to help in curing the patient of his stroke.

Constipation

For all those who suffer from **constipation,** eat one raw onion with buttermilk in every meal and stop worrying about your stomach. This was fed to us with lunch, every summer, so that we did not suffer from sunstroke, either. Naturally, we had to brush our teeth vigorously before going back to school.

Unfortunately, except in Italy and Spain, garlic and raw onion is not an integral part of Western cuisine, which goes by the truthful dictum – *An Apple a day keeps the doctor away, but some garlic, a day, keeps everybody away.* No wonder, so many people suffer from heart disease. If you can manage to swallow three cloves of raw garlic, every night before sleeping, you would be astonished at the fall of your cholesterol level and a lowering of the possibility of your suffering from heart problems. But no, as the finicky lady in your life gets nauseated by the smell of raw garlic emanating from you, you are not going to eat it. Ah, well.

Kidney stones

Powder 25 g of Papaya root. Drink two spoons of this powder in warm water two times a day. This helps in dissolving the kidney stones.

Fresh Apple juice prevents kidney stones from forming.

Adding more almonds to your daily diet prevent your kidney from malfunctioning. Also, you may try this remedy if your kidneys have started to give you problems – powder 2 teaspoons of coriander seeds and steep them in a glass of boiling hot water for 5 min. Add sugar and milk to taste. A frequent intake of this natural remedy is going to get rid of all the toxins accumulated in your kidneys.

Piles Remedy

Here are some more effective natural remedies for **Piles**.

Make sure that you have plenty of lassi with your food. Not only does this treat piles, but it also eradicates it. Add 1/4 teaspoon of a mixture of powdered carom seeds, roasted black cumin seeds, unroasted black cumin seeds and white rock salt to the buttermilk. If you have the fortitude, you would want to mix 3 teaspoons of fresh bitter gourd juice in this buttermilk.

Incidentally, fresh bitter gourd juice is one of the most popular and well-known of natural **Diabetes** cures in India.

People in the East do not suffer much from piles, because they cannot resist eating lots of fresh horseradish. That is because this is the best cure for piles, ever. If you are suffering from a bad case of piles , and you find yourself in an Eastern village, the lady of the house is going to hold you by your nose and force you to drink 1/4 cup of fresh horseradish juice morning and evening until your system gets working normally again.

An aunt of mine told me this remedy which worked for her. Her piles problem came through not eating fresh fruit and vegetables and suffering from constipation. She mixed 1 teaspoon of fresh mint leaves with a 1 teaspoon of honey and 1 teaspoon lemon juice. She gulped this down 3 times a day for around 15 days and there you are, she was cured. Needless to say, fresh fruit and vegetables are now an integral part of her daily diet.

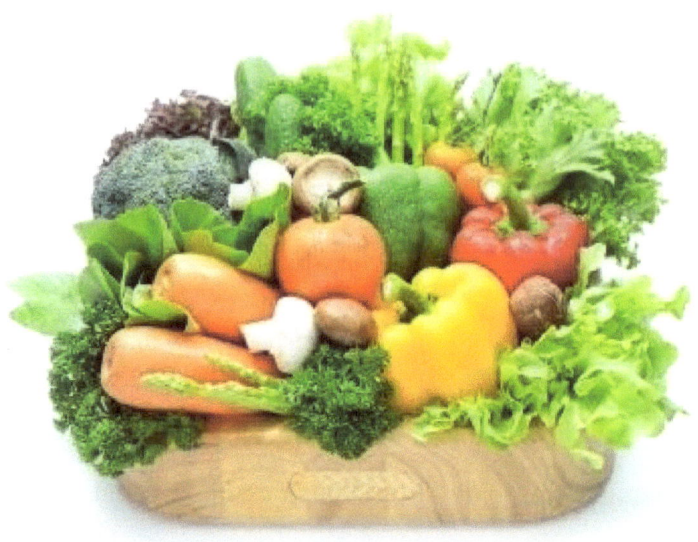

Plenty of greens and roughage- fibers- a day keeps Piles away.

Hair Care

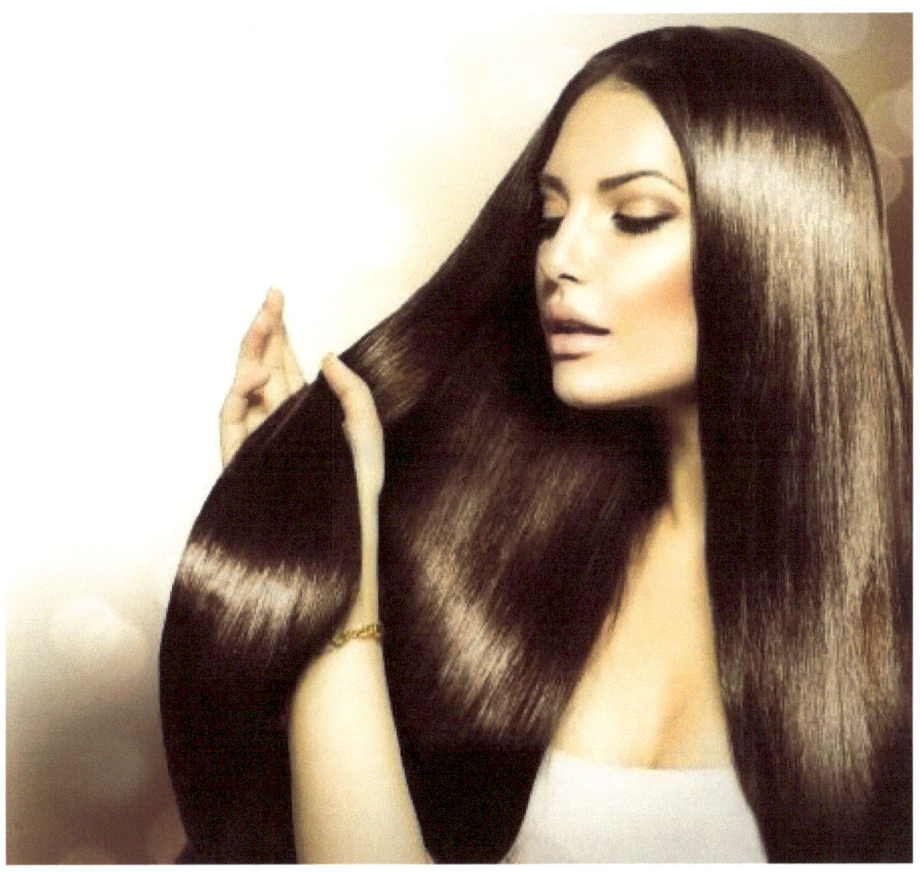

How to Get Rid of Baldness

If the hair follicle is destroyed, there is no question of hair ever growing again. But there is always a chance of a dormant hair follicle being stimulated enough by this recipe.

- Grind raw Amla (gooseberry) in a little yogurt and apply the mixture to your scalp. Leave it on for two hours and then shampoo it. A twice a week application with show you results within a couple of months, if the hair follicle has not been destroyed by heat or sunlight.

Alopecia Areata

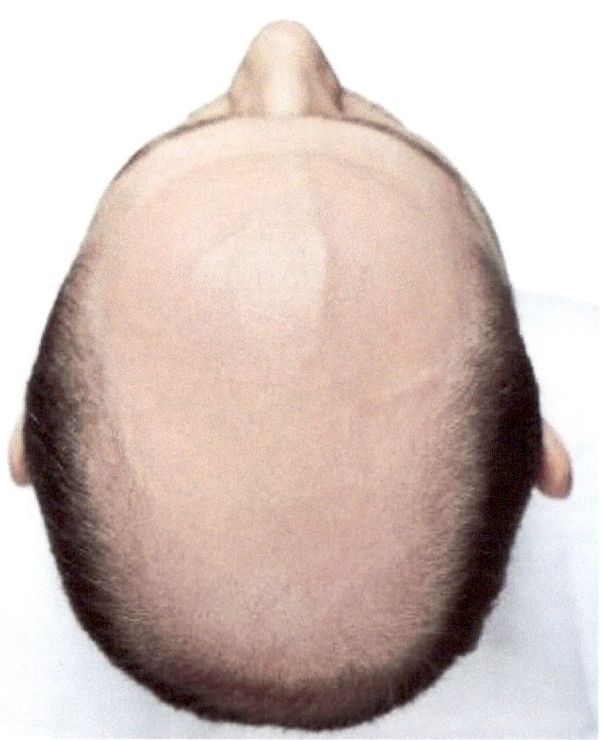

The problem of Alopecia Areata (baldness.)- Ladies are rather lucky, they are not bothered by a shining bald pate which is the bane of so many gentlemen, who do not look as attractive as Yul Brynner. But as there are exceptions to the rule everywhere, I found that there were huge bald patches on my scalp, even though I had a very thick head of hair.

Now,here were we, about eight hours journey away from civilization where this affliction could be treated properly , living deep in the remote and most God forsaken areas of those mysterious, dark jungles of India, thanks to a peripatetic father .So the doctors decided that it was a case of vitamin deficiency and gave me vitamin B injections in my scalp once a week.

This treatment was successful in my case, because I never suffered from Alopecia again, (except when I was at University and I am sure that the unguent given to me by the resident white witch had lots of turpentine oil, desi ghee and other exotic herbs in it. I have never forgiven myself for not taking the recipe from her, but then, I did not know that nearly quarter of a century later I would be compiling a herbarium…

As the injection in the scalp treatment is rather painful, I would give you the Oriental herbal cure for alopecia.

Cassia fistula is a very popular flowering plant. It is called *Amaltas* or Laburnum (Golden Shower). Even though that particular name has unacceptable and crude connotations in the West, it must be understood that we only mean to describe the beautiful hanging flowers of the laburnum!

Collect the bark, flowers, roots and leaves of Cassia. Burn them to an ash and powder them. Then make a paste in goat's or cow's milk and apply it up on the scalp. See the hair growing within a month. I know this remedy works because the people of the Northern villages in the Indian subcontinent have long unshorn hair, and are very rarely bald.

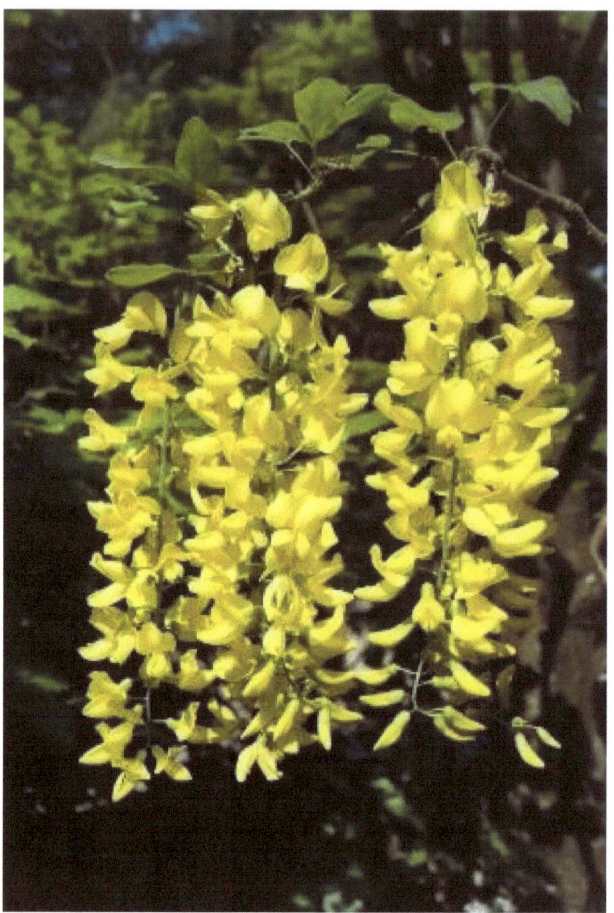

Cassia Flower

Burning to An Ash

This carbonization is normally done in places where you have easy access to wooden charcoal or a mud oven [also called a tandoor.] This was done in ancient times when we did not have high-powered burners so I wonder if it is going to have the same effect if you place them in a seasoned clay container and put them over the kitchen stove fire until they crackle and burn up. No point in not using technology when it is there. After all, we need these items burnt.

This is normally done by placing all these items in a clay earthenware pot. The pot is then sealed with mud with a wet mud paste applied to the sides of the pot so that it does not crack when it is put in the really hot oven. Now place it under burning coals for an hour. When you unseal the pot, you are going to find all the items in it, burnt to a crisp. This is the powder, which is going to be used in herbal remedies.

What on Earth Is Desi Ghee?

Desi Ghee is freshly made butter put onto a slow fire and melted without burning. This is the most powerful basis of any herbal remedy in many parts of the East because of its sheer concentrated natural healing power.

This concentrated clarified butter, is extremely concentrated and a very powerful healing agent. It is normally used in the making up of herbal medicines, because it is made of pure creamy milk butter. It is also used in making beauty creams, potions, lotions and other skin ointments.

It has a powerful aroma, and that is why only just a spoonful is added to fry meats. It is going to float on the surface of the meat dish, after it has been cooked, so you need to stir the gravy before serving. Also, the food is not going to taste greasy, even though it looks like it has been swimming in fat.

Desi ghee is the concentrated form of pure butter, which is heated to reduce the butter of all the impurities as well as moisture. This concentrated butter is normally used in Eastern cuisine, for searing meat, sautéing and frying food, because they offer its higher burning point. You make this at home by taking 2 pounds of best unsalted butter and melting it in a heavy bottomed pan. Allow the butter to liquefy on low heat for about 40 minutes. Maintain this simmering point, until all of the moisture in the butter has evaporated. The impurities are going to sink to the bottom of the pan. Remember to keep stirring the butter, so that it does not burn.

Pour off the clear butter and strain it through several thicknesses of muslin cloth. This butter is going to last for about a year, if it is placed in a cool and dry place. This butter is exorbitantly expensive. So in the East, people with easy access to plenty fresh milk make it right in their kitchens for crisp delicious frying results, and adding that taste of pure butter to all their dishes.

Premature Graying of Hair

Some years ago, one of my good friends Sue Yung, happened to be browsing through the newspaper, and commented on the fact that Mr. George Clooney was worried about his hair going distinguished gray at the tender young age of 49.

Our dialogue went something like this:

Sue (*sniffing*) – Hey man, what's the matter with this guy? (Anybody who imagines that Chinese speak likee thisee had better drag themselves into the 21st century.) He's worried about his hair growing prematurely gray at the age of 49 and wants to know how to stop this premature graying. Hasn't he heard about nature taking its own course?

I – (*talking like a TV anchor)* –Yerss, isn't it amayr-zing?

Sue - Well, we have to give the poor guy some sympathy. When a bewildered force such as he is pursued by every red blooded dame out there you can be sure, as long as you live, something's gotta give, something's gotta give, something's gotta give. And in this case, the hair have caught the brunt of that stunt. Tough luck!

I—(*with lots of ghastly sprightliness, still in TV anchor mode.*)—So why does he not turn suicide blond and have done with it? All he would ever have to bother about, then, would be the choice between ash blond, medium blond or sunbleached blond, Baywatch blond or James Blond.

Sue does not like this idea, after all, all brunettes should stick together and think of some solution for the premature graying of hair. And so, thanks to Chinese pressure points, here is the solution for the **premature graying of hair.**

How to darken your hair naturally

Fist up your palms. Place them together and start rubbing your nails against each other. Move both hands. Ladies will please not rub their thumbnails unless they want to be known as the bearded lady. But any teenaged youngster who is bothered about a thin growth of facial hair can use this rubbing your thumbnails method to make sure that nobody is going to look askance at him and wonder if he needs any hormone treatment.

How do I know this method works? The proof of the pudding is my mother, whose below knee length hair suddenly started to turn gray, when she hit her 60s. [She is 73, now, and a proud grandma in her turn with salt and pepper hair.] Five to 10 minutes of rubbing her nails together, whenever she had the time, showed an astonishing growth of black patches among the silver. Her hair is now turning black naturally and there is no question of her using any dyeing agents ever.

I noticed the same nail rubbing being done by females sitting in the winter sun on the grass and gossiping. Good way to keep your hair black, while you are dissecting reputations and pay packages.

Another effective way to stop graying of hair and hair loss is a regular massage of the scalp and hair with lime juice.

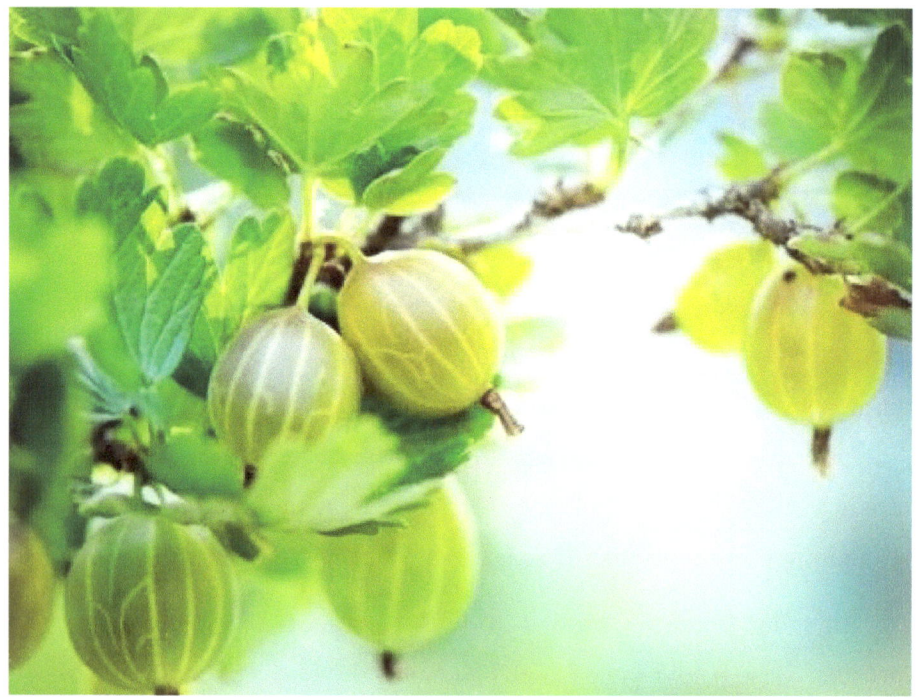

Gooseberries are excellent for hair care

But Sue happens to be really adamant about the most effective way of making sure that Mr. Clooney stops worrying about future graying of hair. For that he can get an assurance that the following remedies are also very effective. And if they do not work, I will take on the dare, and change my name to something idiotic like   Intipinti Papatinti like any imaginative budding and would be rockstar so that I have a thorough excuse to act thoroughly IQ room temperature, frivolous, tiresome, silly and spoiled brattish!

Make a mixture of Amla (*Emblica officianalis* powder) in freshly squeezed lime juice. Massage your scalp with this mixture. Not only will it prevent hair from growing gray, but it will ensure that hair loss is also drastically reduced.

Mehndi (*Henna _ Lawrensia*) has long been known as a natural hair conditioner to everyone in the Orient. But because it gives the hair a reddish tinge, I am going to give you a recipe to reduce the auburn qualities of Henna.

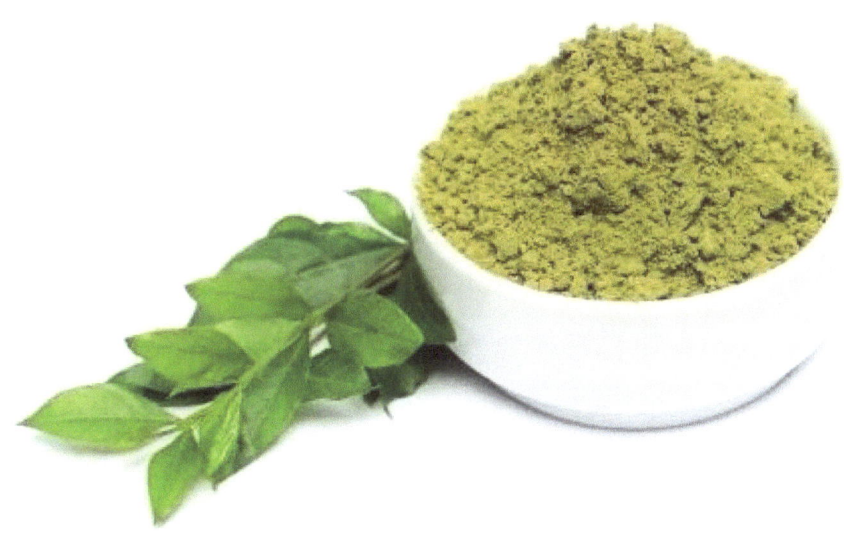

Gather some fresh leaves of Henna. Add them to 200 g of milk . Add five tablespoons of powdered *Amla [Gooseberry]* to this mixture. Bring this to a boil. Apply the milk/ Amla /henna extract paste to your hair. Wash your hair with water in which you soaked some dried gooseberries overnight. This procedure has to be done twice a week to get the best results . This is the most effective way to darken your hair at the roots.

Gooseberry Oil

To make sure that your hair remained dark, do not use any artificial chemical-based conditioner on them. Instead, use gooseberry oil.

To make this oil, you need to put equal amounts of raw Gooseberry in sesame oil. Place this in the sun for 15 days. This slow cooking of this oil and the gooseberries is going to make a powerful oil concentrate. Now filter the oil and put it in a glass bottle. This prevents your hair from growing white, even though you grow old, premature grayness, soft, long and silky. So if you have ever admired the long beautiful hair of the Oriental lady, she may or may not tell you her secret – gooseberry oil!

This oil is applied to the hair, after you have shampooed it twice a week. Try it out right now, and you are going to see your hair growing sleek, shiny, well-managed, and healthy within two months.

Preventing Hair Loss

In the same way, this recipe was given to me by a lady who is in her 70s, but managed to prevent hair loss with the help of gooseberries.

Take equal amounts of henna powder and Gooseberry powder. Soak them in water, and make a paste. Apply this paste on all of your hair and on your scalp and leave on for four hours. After that wash your hair with plain water [no shampoo or soap.] When your hair is dry, apply the Gooseberry hair oil.

This is going to give your hair a natural dark sheen. Do this once a week and you are soon going to see your hair, changing color to its natural color from gray, as well as preventing excessive hair loss.

Asvhagandha

http://en.wikipedia.org/wiki/Withania_somnifera

It was only in the late 20th century that the West got to know about the miracle plant known as **Ashvagandha (Withania somnifera)**. It has been known since ancient times to cure **leuchorrhea, impotence** and one could almost call it the Eastern natural equivalent to Viagra.

Being a rather introvertish female, I was rather shy at first about asking the recipe for this potent remedy of a herbalist, but well, here it is.

250 grams *Nagori ashwagandha* (that is its real ancient name), 250 g dried ginger (*saunth*). Powder, mix together and filter it . Then take enough of desi ghee for frying it. Fry this mixture until it is dark brown. Then add 250 g of molasses (*khand*) and enough of water and fry until the ghee rises to the surface. 10 grams of this very powerful medicine in 125 g of cow's milk is what make the earthy rustic women of the North proudly describe their husbands as bulls.

Reminds me of Santino's wife boasting about her husband in *The Godfather.* And that made one silly female go straight up to him and demand proof. Limits of stupidity, I think, but Women Will Be Women. And many will act in perverse ways.

I gave this recipe to a Spanish friend of mine, and he was extremely pleased with it. When he asked me to make up another package for him, I refused point-blank. I would rather not have people indulging in ancient potency enhancing recipes, because that exposes you to a variety of ills. Overindulgence in this activity is going to bring about possible physical debilitation. So be very careful and do not act Men Will Be Men, and give the proof to all and sundry.

Remember that there are plenty of social diseases prevalent in society, but still if you will not listen to good sense and are careless, you can cure **Gonorrhea** by roasting one gram alum and 1 g Mishri (extremely pure crystallized sugar/rock candy) . Powder this mixture and drink it in 125 g water for one week. This is an ancient soldiers cure, because they were the people who used to be most exposed to social diseases, thanks to their careless mode of living, while soldiering in new lands.

Asthma

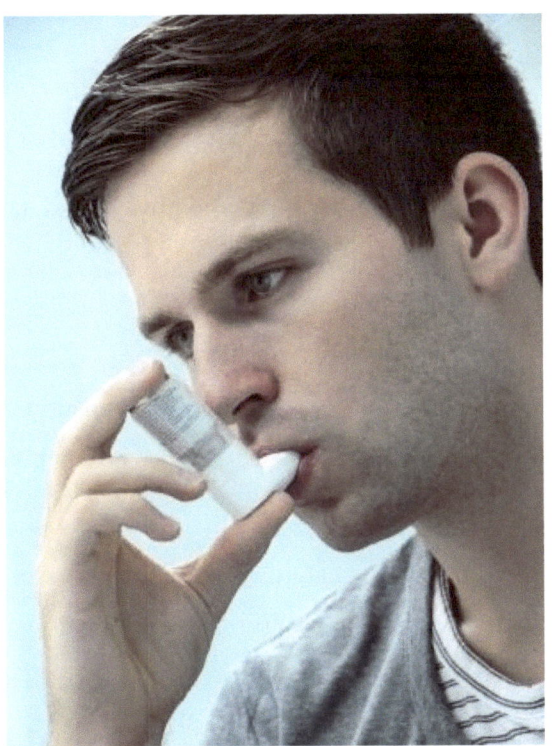

The magical plant Ashwagandha also cures **Bronchitis and asthma in 10 days! (Why oh why are people suffering when they can have such herbal remedies at their fingertips? Anyway, read on...)**

Add 250 g powdered Aswagandha to desi ghee. Use the above recipe to make a fried desi ghee- aswagandha mixture to make up a mixture which has to be drunk with milk once a day until the bronchitis/ asthma is cured.

This mixture taken just before you go to sleep can also cure **insomnia.**

Apart from this, asthma can be cured by the following recipe. It is a 3 times a day into 15 days course.

1 g Powdered bay leaf

10 g honey

125 g goat's milk

Drink this, three times a day for 15 days, and get rid of that **asthma.** If you cannot find goats anywhere, you could always find dates.

250 g dates

Hundred grams black pepper.

Roast them together. The dates have to be chopped in small pieces, so that you can make pellets. Drink down 1 pellet with hot milk, two times a day.

You can also cure **Asthma** naturally by mixing 1 teaspoon of honey with half a teaspoon of cinnamon powder and washing down with warm milk, every night.

Are you suffering from the **Early Stages of Asthma**?

Boil 10 cloves of fresh garlic in half a cup of milk. Drink this down every night. This is going to give you excellent results in the early stages of asthma.

Here is another very effective remedy for asthma, which has come down through the ages – boil 6 cloves in just 3 teaspoons of water. Remove the cloves and add this concentrated powerful expectorant to 1 teaspoon of honey. Drink it down 3 times a day.

What Is the Best Diet for a Person Suffering from Asthma?

- Stop eating rice altogether, especially at dinnertime.

- Dairy products aggravate asthma. So stop drinking milk and eating dairy products.

- No citrus fruits, please. Also, no cold drinks, spicy and greasy deep-fried food or ice creams.

- Add apples, watermelon, and more fresh fruit and vegetables to your diet.

- Try drinking 1 teaspoon of honey in a glass of hot water before you go to sleep. This is going to keep your throat passage irrigated while you rest. It prevents the accumulation of phlegm.

Sciatica Remedy

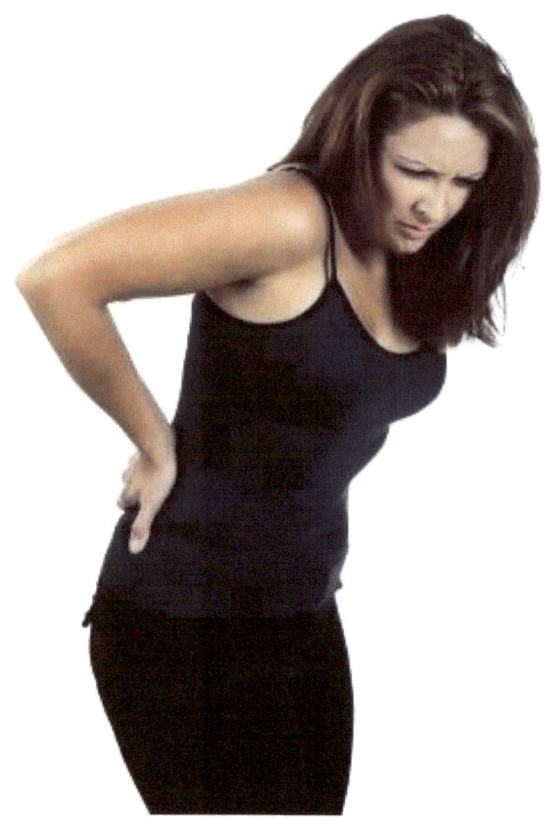

Take equal amounts of dried neem tree bark, ashvagandha powder, dried ginger powder and long pepper(pippalamool) powder. Grind these up and bottle them. Now you are going to drink one teaspoonful of this mixture twice every day with milk. This remedy has long been in use in the East, and is normally used to cure people in the mountains, who were exposed to the cold and are not suffering from muscular camps in the leg.

You may also want to massage that affected area with two cloves of garlic burnt in some sesame oil. Filter this oil and massage that affected area four times a day. This is going to ease the muscles and pain.

Knowing about Hot and Cold Foods

This knowledge of the type of foods – hot and cold – has come down from the ages in the East, and even though there is no scientific backing behind it, everyone in the East understands when somebody says that one should not eat a hot food or a cold food. This has nothing to do with the temperature of the food or its attractive and overall seductive gorgeousness – which is the common slang to describe the word "hot"! Instead, it has everything to do with its essential "nature".

So when you are suffering from Sciatica you do not eat cool foods.

Let me explain in language which even I can understand without getting thoroughly confused!

These are things which you need to avoid when you are suffering from painful Sciatica. Do not eat citric fruit like lemons, oranges and limes. They are considered to be cold and promote Sciatica. That is why you can eat them as much as you like in summer, but they are not advised in the winter.

Mangoes are considered to be "hot", and that is why too many mangoes in summer will cause a nosebleed. That is why mangoes are normally placed in a bucket of cold water, and allowed to "cool down," before they are fed to hungry humans on a hot summer day.

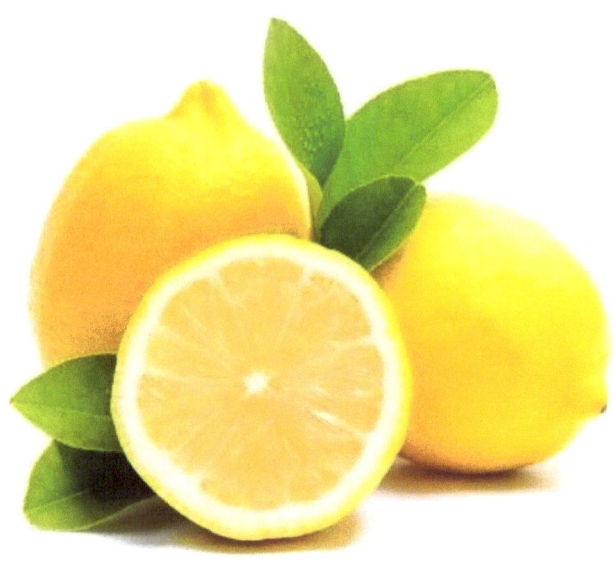

Lemons and other citric fruits should be avoided as far as possible in the winter.

Pomegranates and guavas are also not advised. Sour pickles and chutneys, especially those made up of tomatoes and tamarind are also to be removed from your diet, along with radish, yogurt and turnips.

Instead, eat more proteins, fish, spices, eggs and foods considered to be "hot. "In 21st century parley, translated from second century parley, hot food items include cloves, cardamoms, cinnamon, meat products, egg products, nuts and dry fruits like walnuts, cashews, raisins, and other foodstuffs which you consider difficult to digest in summer. These are "hot" foods. Anything easily digestible in summer are "cold" foods. These include all the other easily available summer vegetables. You do not eat them in winter. [Unless of course, you have an easily accessible all year around cold storage, thanks to which you can eat peas and spinach in the summer, – bad call – and cucumbers, watermelons and gourds in the winter.]

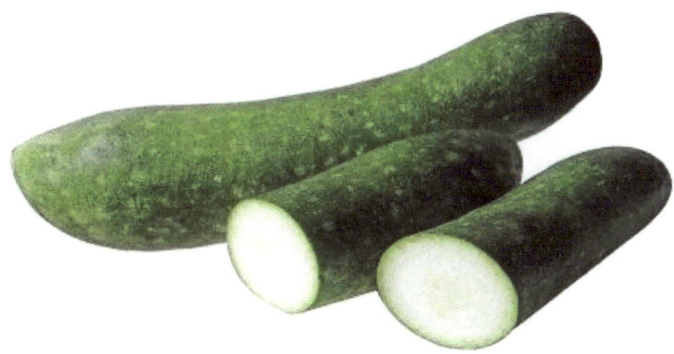

For people who want to know more about this Oriental concept, I found the information given on this site very useful. You may want to look at it. This idea is just not restricted to China, it is also followed in the Middle East, Persia, Egypt, India, and any other Eastern Asian civilizations of which you could think. The West is waking up to this concept of healthy eating brought down to you since ancient times.

http://www.scottsdaleacupuncture.com/food.htm

Bacopa Scrophulariaceae-Bhrahmi Booti

http://bestbrahmi.com/aboutbrahmi.html

Now let me tell you about one more very important magic herb Brahmi booti. Just like Ashvagandha, this herb is getting to be more and more well-known as a natural curative with powers still unresearched and documented by researchers in the West, but which have been known for millenniums in the East.

Apart from using this herbal powder in herbal gooseberry and soap, nut-based shampoos to prevent hair loss, I am going to use this powder to improve my memory. This is also very good amnesia cure. Drink this when you are in your 40s and 50s and **never bother about Alzheimers ever again.**

- **20 g Bhrahmi booti powder**

- **Six tablespoons almond oil**

- **3 g pepper**

- **3 g crushed cardamom seeds**

Mix these ingredients together. Now this happens to be a very powerful medicine. So you have to drink just the amount which you put upon two pinheads (.22 grams!) with milk every morning and see your memory improving by leaps and bounds.

Fresh sheep liver is also excellent for curing **Memory Loss.**

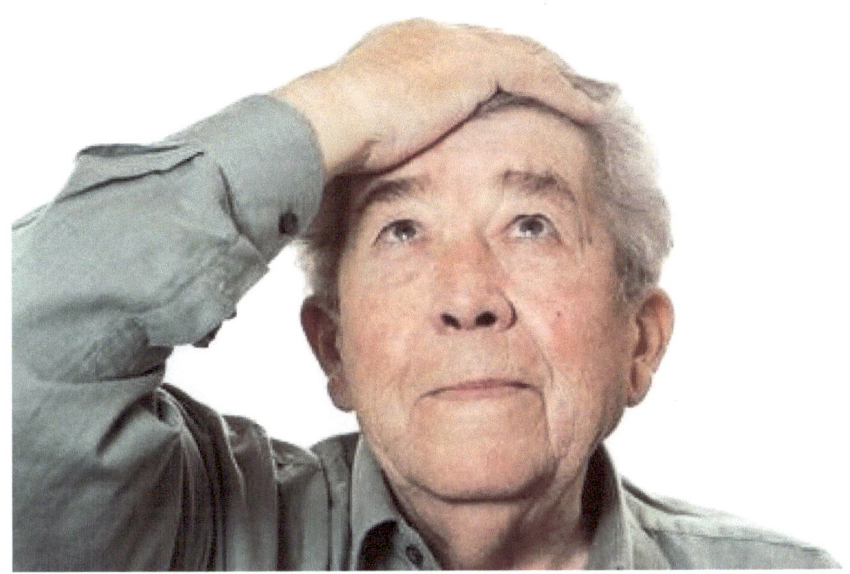

Memory loss or a failing memory is definitely not restricted to the oldest generation. It can occur even in children and young adults.

Epilepsy

Brahmi booti also cures Epilepsy completely

- 10 g of Bhrami juice taken with 10 g of honey for 15 days will cure epilepsy completely.

There is also an exotic surefire cure for epileptics .

- Burn five bedbugs on red-hot coals and make the patient inhale the fumes!

When I spoke about this recipe to a very kind --and logical—writer friend,- who was instrumental in giving me the suggestion of compiling all of my recipes,- she immediately caught the practical point that any epileptic patient would come out of his fit, by the time you hunted out five bedbugs and got the coals to burn red hot!(*(The laughs in this para are all due to Mary Jo Putney. Thank you, Tiger Lady…)*

I agree with her completely. But then, these were the cures which were used in ancient times, when coals were kept burning throughout the day and bedbugs were present a-plenty. This cure was about as drastic as taking off one of your shoes and making the victim inhale the leather, a practice which is still followed in the East today, and is about as efficient as making swooning Victorian ladies constricted by their tight stays and corsets, smell burnt feathers or Sal volatile to get them out of their highbred and languishing fits.

Get Rid Of Bedbugs

And well, if you managed to find the bedbugs (!), it is time to get rid of them by using grandma's time-tested remedy of dissolving 10 g of alum in 250 g of boiling water and then treating your furniture, nooks, crevices, and crannies to this solution.

http://www.123rf.com/photo_14545159_cockroach-sign.html

Make your house cockroach free

In the same manner, you could get rid of all the **cockroaches** in the house by making pellets of wheat flour with soda bicarbonate and scattering them in cockroach infested places. This does not kill them, but renders them incapable of multiplying. Beats poisonous and toxic boric acid, every time. I place these pellets around areas where cockroaches can get easy access to water. Especially the bathroom and kitchen drain. Try it out right now.

Ear Infections

Thanks to living in an insalubrious wet countryside and staying under water in the swimming pool/pond in our garden four hours out of the 24 allotted to us every day without fail, I used to suffer a lot from ear infections, (*Otitis externa*) as a child. This meant a regular visit to the doctor every three days to remove the horrible fungal growth and painful discharge. [But would I leave off swimming, certainly not. Everything else was responsible for my ear aching so much. The continuous rain, the carelessness of the doctor, ear wax…]

Until one day granny got really fed up by my yowling and howling and made up this home remedy.

Garlic Remedy

Three cloves ground garlic boiled in 50 g mustard oil. Two drops twice a day in my ear at night and then cleaning with an earbud next morning cleared up the infection within a week, never to return again!

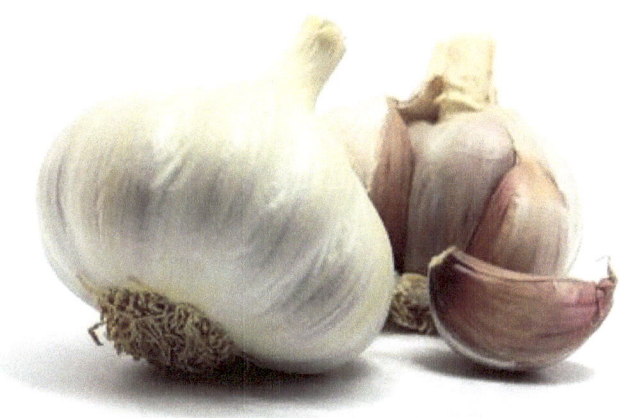

Granny did not have an important ingredient, which is known as sindoor or Kumkum, (10 grams ,) but even so, the recipe worked.

This mixture of mustard oil, ground garlic and sindoor is the basis of many ear cures in the East, even today.

This bright red powder is considered to be a very precious part of every Indian Hindu bride's beauty box. It is also used in the Hindu religious ceremonies.

Kum Kum

What is the significance of this bright vermilion powder in India?

In every Hindu religious ceremony, a bright vermilion powder known as kumkum is applied upon the forehead of the worshipers to signify that they have been blessed by the gods. When the same powder is applied by a man upon the forehead hair parting of a woman, it signifies that she is now wed to him. From then on, the woman is going to show her marital status by wearing a bright red bindi on her forehead, and a red streak in her hair parting which will be now known as Sindoor and not kum-kum.

Let me tell you about the significance of sindoor. I know a lady who is born a Hindu but is happily married in an inter-religious marriage. She asked her newlywed husband to apply Sindoor on her forehead, during the marriage ceremony. This meant that they would be together till death did them part and the red of happiness would follow them throughout their lives, according to the vows that they had taken in the presence of God. He did so, – even though this ritual is not part of his own particular religious marriage ceremony – and then brought his newly wedded wife to get the blessings of all the family members.

Some years later, I noticed her one morning stumbling with eyes closed to the bathroom where she immediately placed a pinch of red sindoor on her forehead, bowed her folded hands, and prayed for the well-being of her husband and children and *then* opened her eyes to see her face in the mirror, first thing in the morning.

Her explanation to my querying look was that the status of a Hindu widow in India was that she did not wear any red signifying happiness. That is why she did not wear sindoor on her forehead.

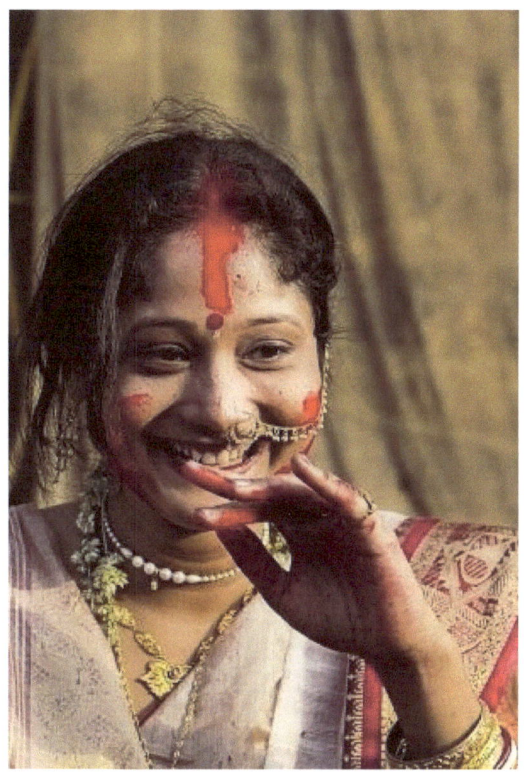

During the Bengali religious festival of Durga Puja, married women not only apply sindoor to their foreheads, but also to their faces to signify happiness.

That lady did not want her eyes to ever see her forehead unadorned with the red sindoor of marriage, *even by mistake, or through sheer negligence and carelessness, being a good and traditionally brought up wife.* That is why she kept her eyes shut, before looking in the mirror in the morning.

I found out later, that this is a part of every Hindu wife's waking up morning ritual, coming down from the ages.

This tradition of showing your happiness in your marital state has come down to ancient times and is an integral part of every Hindu marriage.

Anyway, here is the recipe for how to make **natural sindoor/Kumkum** at home.

The one that you get in the market is going to be made up of powdered lead oxide to give it that deep red color. That is why, that can definitely not be sprinkled on open wounds to stop the bleeding. However, this was done with homemade powder, and it was alum and turmeric, which stopped the bleeding.

Add hundred grams of powdered slaked lime to hundred grams of turmeric and 10 grams of powdered alum. Put it on high heat, and keep adding little amounts of water till the chemical reaction turns the powder completely red. Here is your beautiful kumkum which is ready for application after filtering. So if you want to adorn your forehead with a dark red traditional Eastern powder, – this was part of the fashion scene during the 60s flower child movement – go on right ahead!

Periodic Deafness can be treated by burning 8 cloves of garlic in 50 g of sesame oil. Two drops a day will cure periodic deafness.

Conclusion

In this eclectic mixture of information, remedies, recipes and traditional knowledge, you have learned something of the ancient culture and tradition of the East. The East has this knowledge passed down through word of mouth, for millenniums, and as writing was not done during the prehistoric age, teachers used their students'retentive and brain power to instill knowledge in them which would be passed on to future generations. This memory, of course, was enhanced by a diet supplement consisting of gooseberries and bhrahmi booti, which are still being used as a memory enhancer in the East today.

Most of this word-of-mouth got lost in the translation, and was forgotten until man learned how to write on clay tablets, dried leaves and papyri. They also made up future religious textbooks.

These precious manuscripts are now being studied, so that the wisdom of the ancients can be passed down to us. But because we belong to a cynical age, we do not take everything for gospel truth. And we should not do so. Because most of these cures, we know are placebos, especially those accompanied with chanting and the placing of animal bones or other herbs on affected parts of the body to get rid of pain.

So you may say, how did people manage to get cured when half of the remedies were quack remedies? Aha, there is the catch. These ancient wise men knew that their remedies were effective. That was because they had already experimented on human guinea pigs with different herbal combinations, through the ages, and then they found the right solution in combination, they noted it down. Nevertheless, they knew all about human beings. Give a human a medicine, and tell him to eat it three times a day, and he is definitely going to feel "cheated" subconsciously. He is going to say to himself, "Is that all, to cure my ailment? Just this silly medicine combination?" And most possibly, he would neglect to eat it or use it because he could not care less.

On the other hand, if the doctor said in very grave and serious tones, fingering his gray beard in a very solemn manner, "Well, your skin ailment is rather complicated and it can only be cured, if you wake up in the morning, bow to the sun Three times, put some neem water leaves in water, leave it for 20 minutes, raise it to the sun, all the while chanting a prayer to the sun god to make your skin as bright and blemish free, as his own radiant face, and then have a bath with that water. Be careful not to talk during all this while, because the sun God is going to be doing his magic, which is going to be interrupted if you open your big mouth. Do this for a whole week and you are definitely going to be blessed by the sun God."

Notice the difference with a little bit of imaginative spiel? This superfluous mumbo-jumbo would impress a human being more, because that showed that the doctor was very knowledgeable and he knew all about talking to the gods and asking their blessings. However, you can see that the cure is in the neem leaves and in the water.

These doctors were the first showmen in the medical world.

However, this was also how superstition, and mumbo-jumbo started and began passing down through the ages until people began to use those chants and quack remedies in lieu of other more useful instructions. That is why, they would rather a witch doctor beat them with neem leaves to get rid of the devils which affected their skin, instead of using the neem leaves in a water solution applied on the skin. And the witch doctor was nothing loth to do so.

He knew all about his importance in the tribe, and he added some of his own mumbo-jumbo to the rituals. And so the generations got more steeped in superstitions, quack remedies and foolish rituals, instead of taking advantage of real honest-to-goodness herbal remedies.

Grandma's natural remedies, however, has all the mumbo-jumbo removed, and these are time-tested remedies. However, if you do not think of them showy enough, *listen, thee, very carefully [slow low tones.] Drinkst thou the fresh juice of one orange every day, without fail, while facing the sun. After that, lift thine arms towards the sun, and touch the ground.*

I can continue in this manner, ad infinitum, and that is what the ancients did, using a mixture of psychology, and experienced knowledge to instill awe in the minds of their listeners. And so it has been done down the centuries.

Anybody reading Lord Dunsany's books about Jorkens is going to be amused at that particular character's way of treating sick people in Arabia. He just had some Epsom salts in his medical box. But he accompanied a dose of Epsom salts with loud incantations, and weird noises which impressed his patients even more and gave him the reputation of being a great knowledgeable and powerful *Hakim.* And so it has been done in the Orient through millenniums.

So, look out for more grandma's natural remedies, with more cures, advice, psychology, and time-tested recipes to keep you healthy throughout your life!

Author Bio

Dueep Jyot Singh is a Management and IT Professional who managed to gather Postgraduate qualifications in Management and English and Degrees in Science, French and Education while pursuing different enjoyable career options like being an hospital administrator, IT,SEO and HRD Database Manager/ trainer, movie scriptwriter, theatre artiste and public speaker, lecturer in French, Marketing and Advertising, ex-Editor of Hearts On Fire (now known as Solctice) Books Missouri USA, advice columnist and cartoonist, publisher and Aviation School trainer, ex- moderator on Medico.in, banker, student councilor ,travelogue writer … among other things! One fine morning, she decided that she had enough of killing herself by Degrees and went back to her first love -- writing. It's more enjoyable! She already has 48 published academic and 14 fiction- in- different- genre books under her belt.

When she is not designing websites or making Graphic design illustrations for clients …including R.L. Stevenson, O.Henry, Dornford Yates, Maurice Walsh, C.N.Williamson, Sapper, Bartimeus and the crown of her collection- Dickens "The Old Curiosity Shop," and so on… Just call her "Renaissance Woman" - collecting herbal remedies, acting like Universal Helping Hand/Agony Aunt, or escaping to her dear mountains for a bit of exploring, collecting herbs and plants, and trekking.

Check out some of the other JD-Biz Publishing books

Gardening Series on Amazon

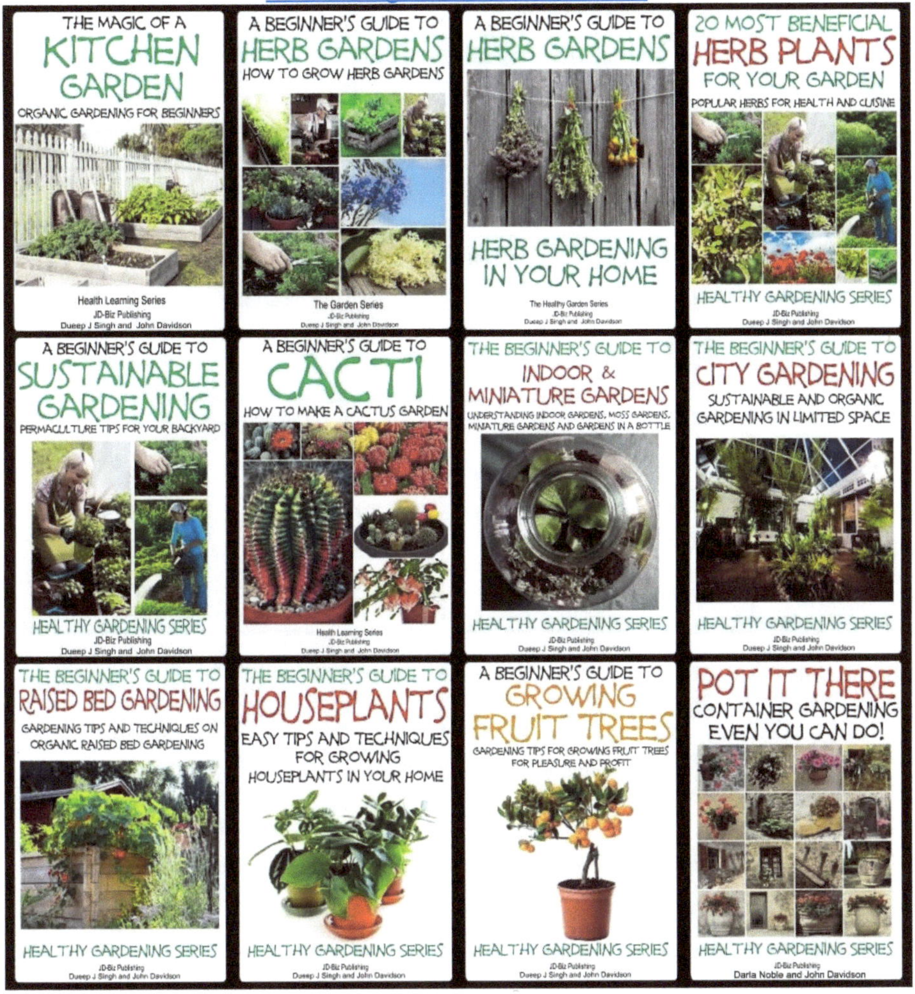

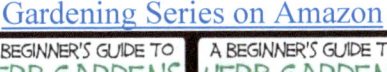

Download Free Books!

http://MendonCottageBooks.com

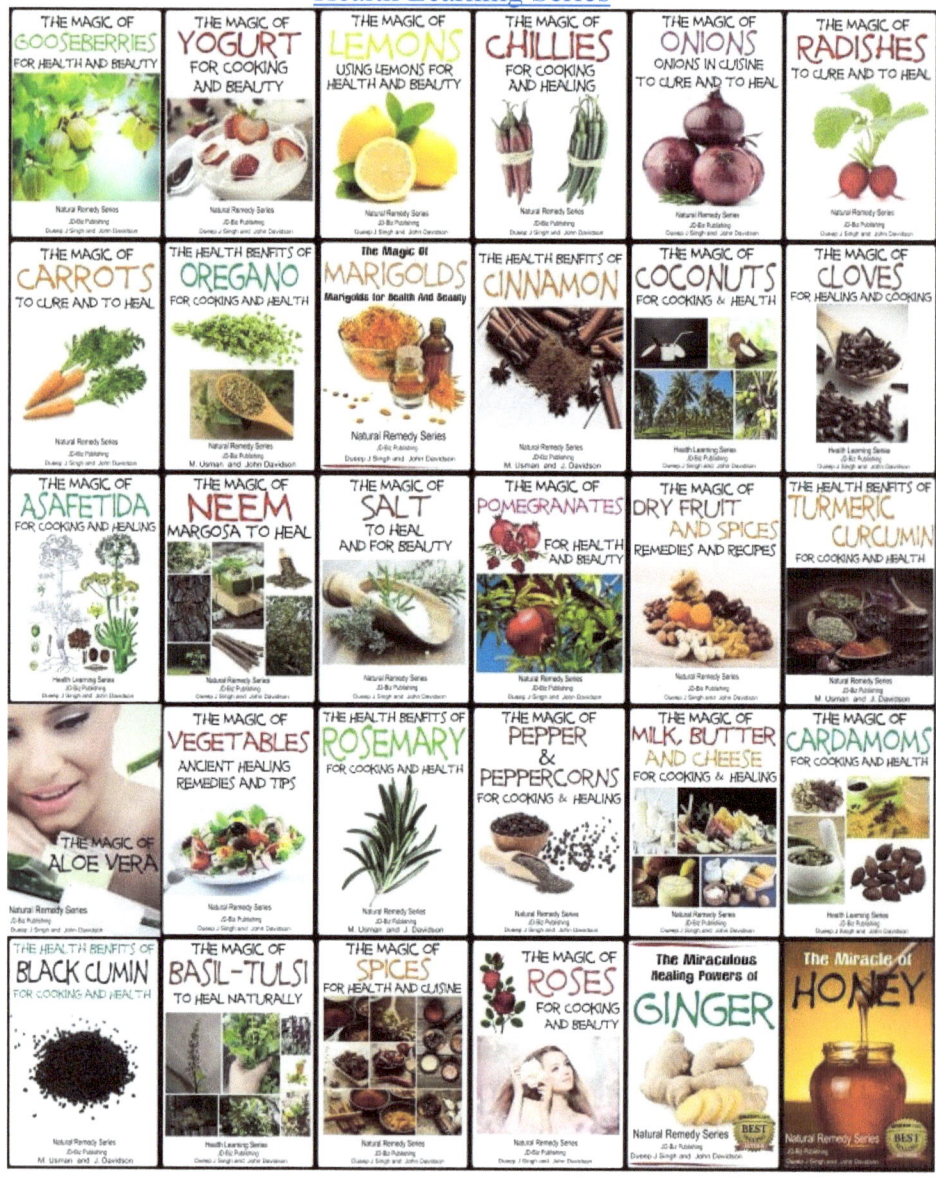

Country Life Books

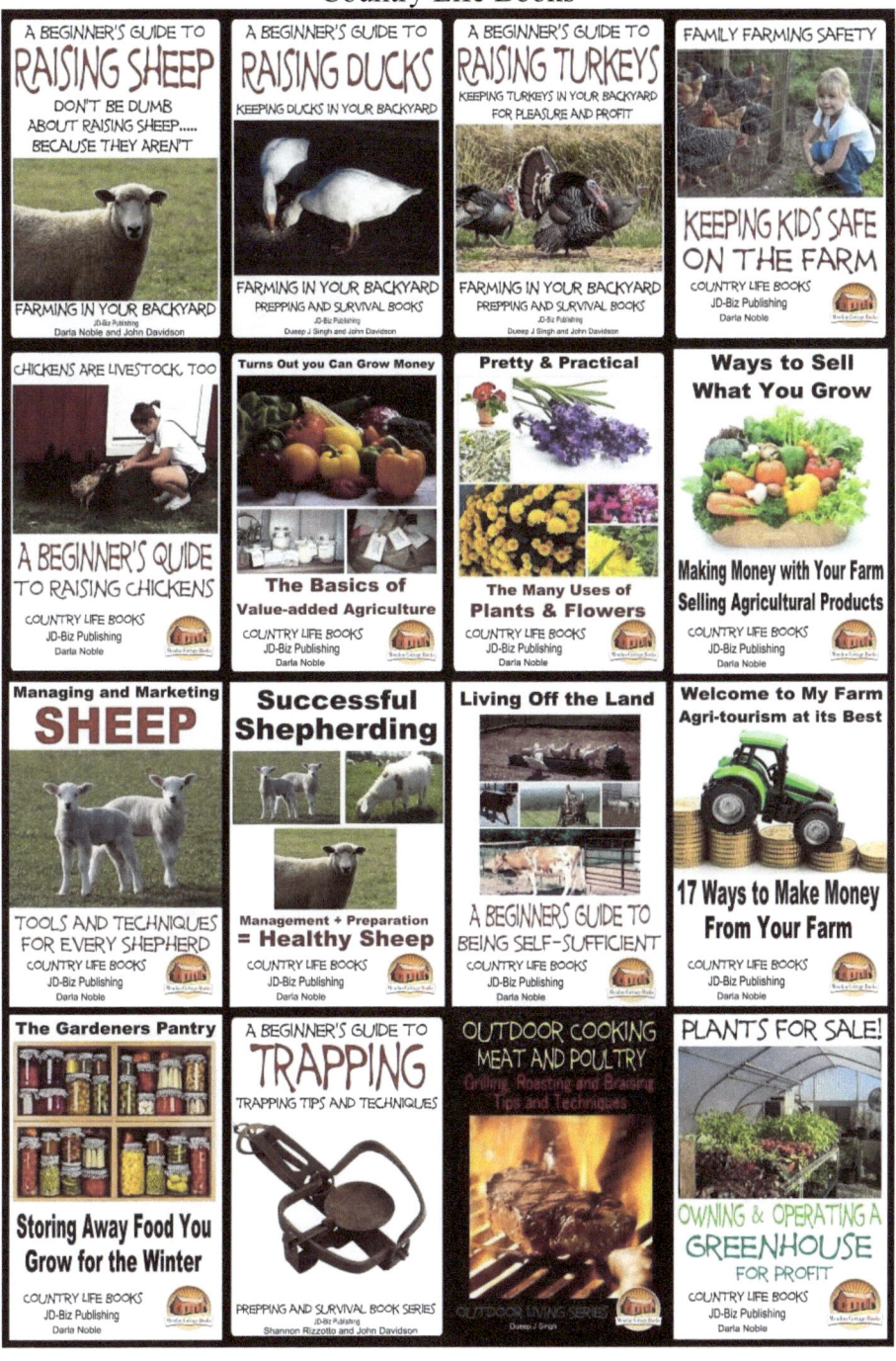

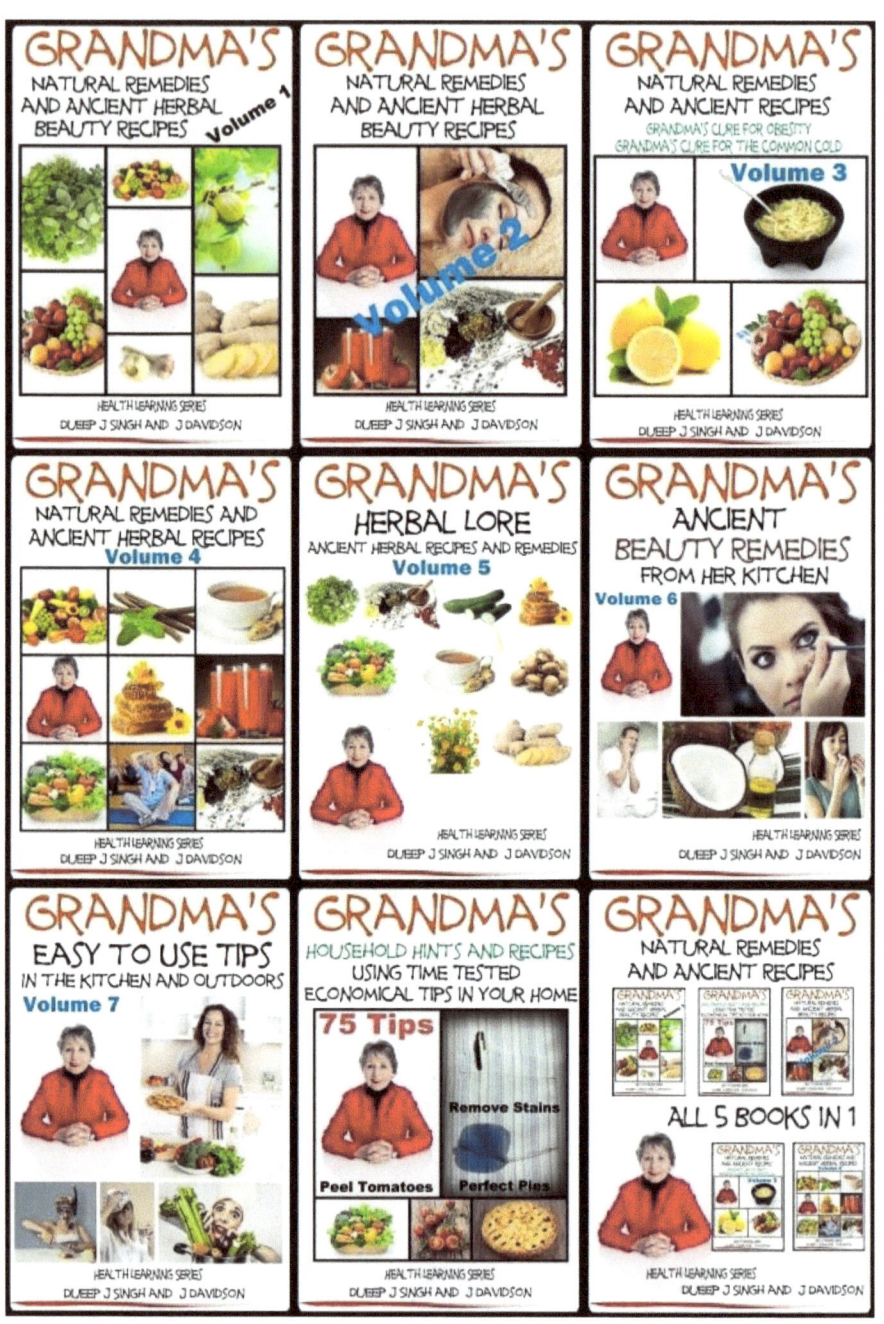

Health Learning Series

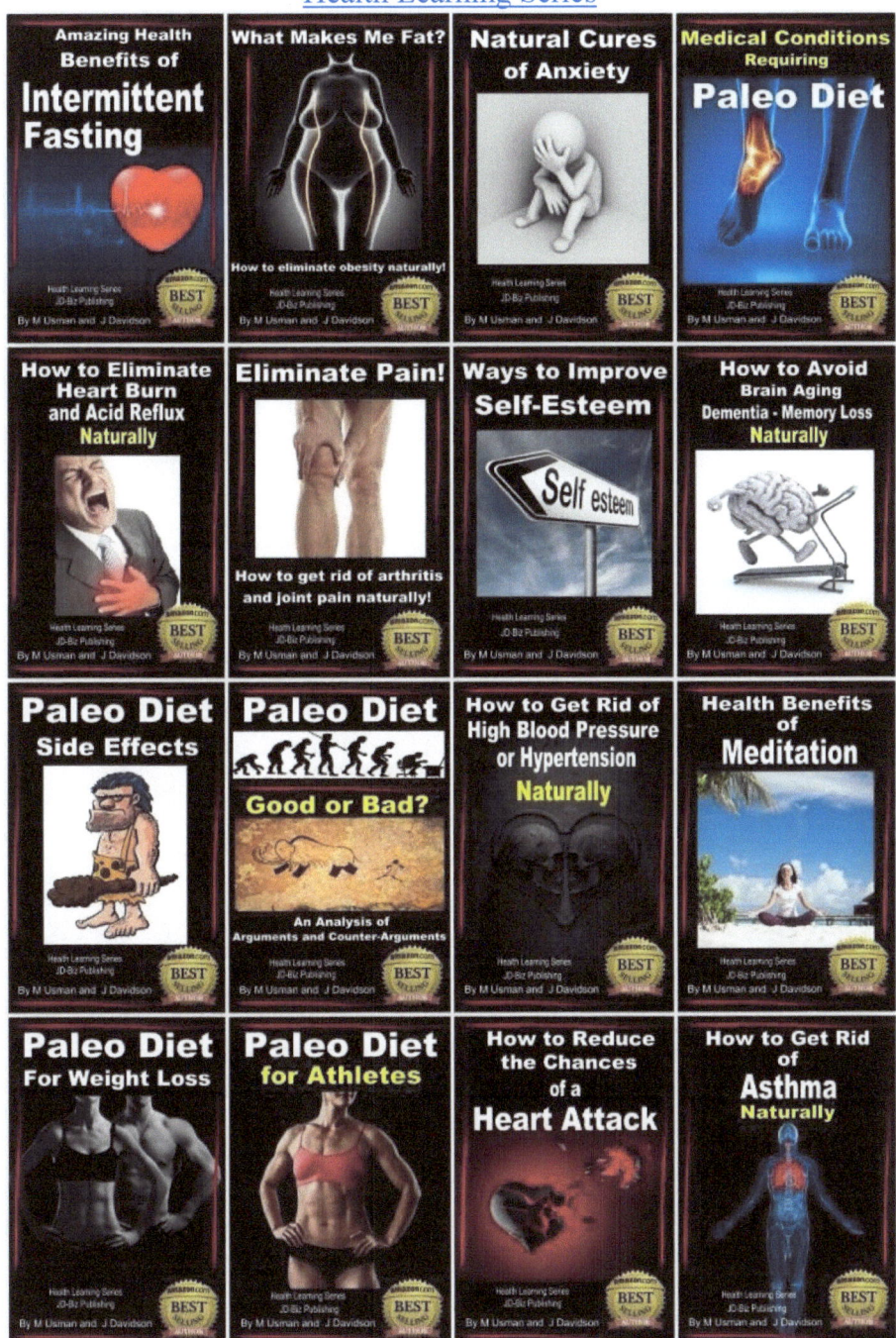

Amazing Animal Book Series

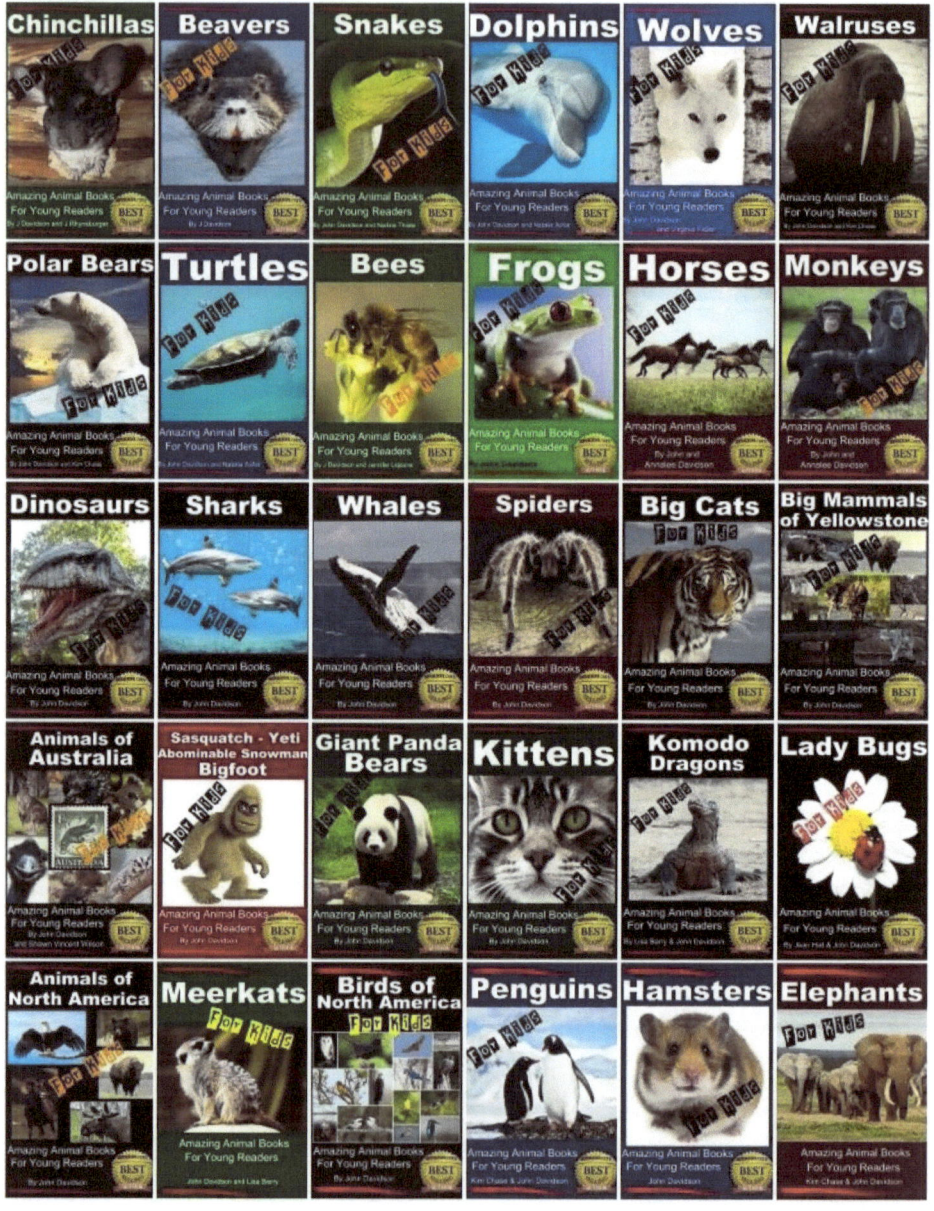

Learn To Draw Series

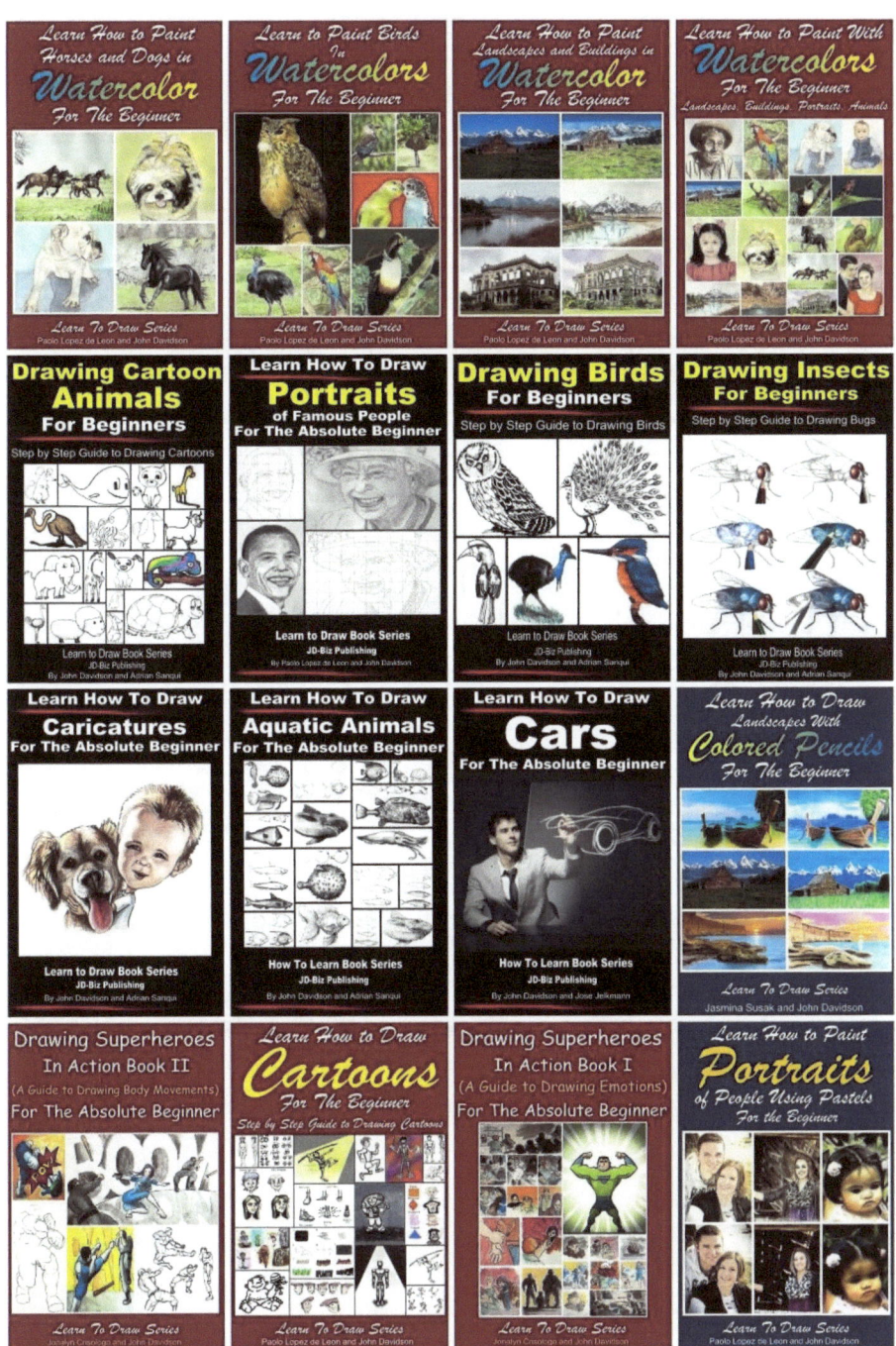

How to Build and Plan Books

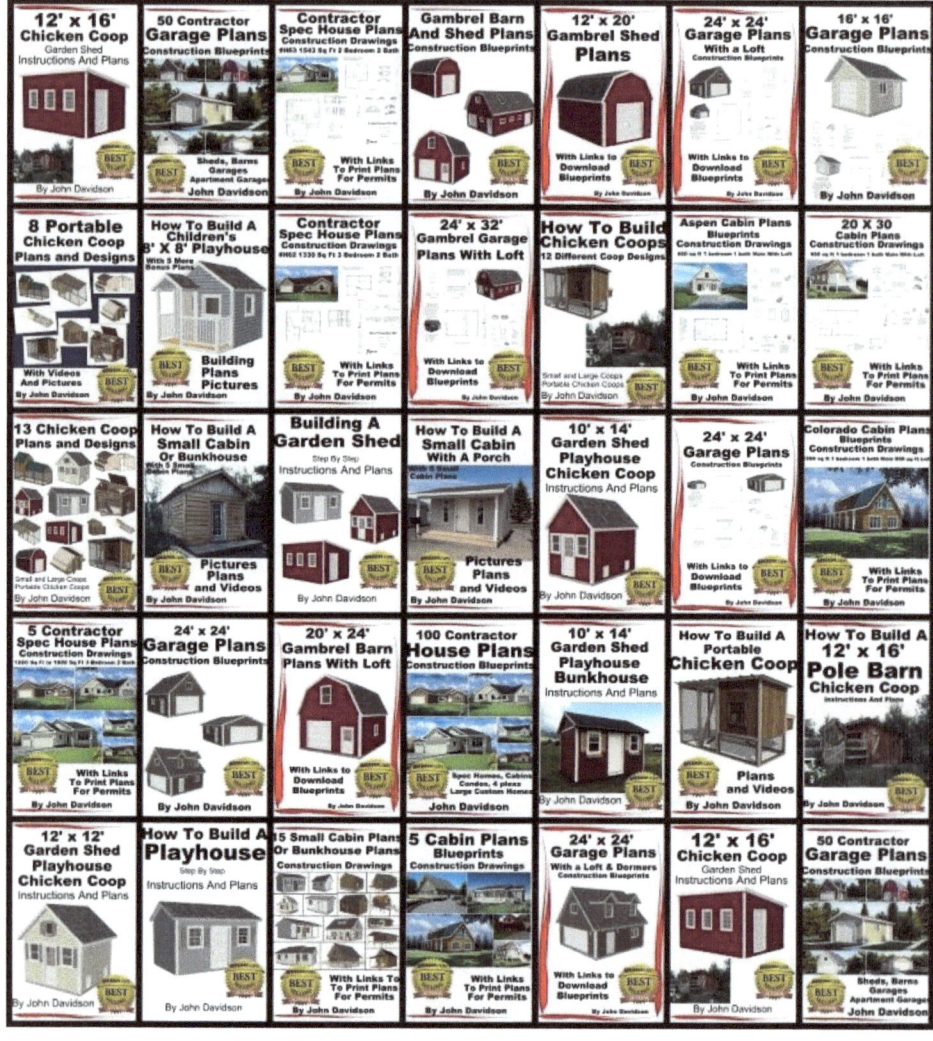

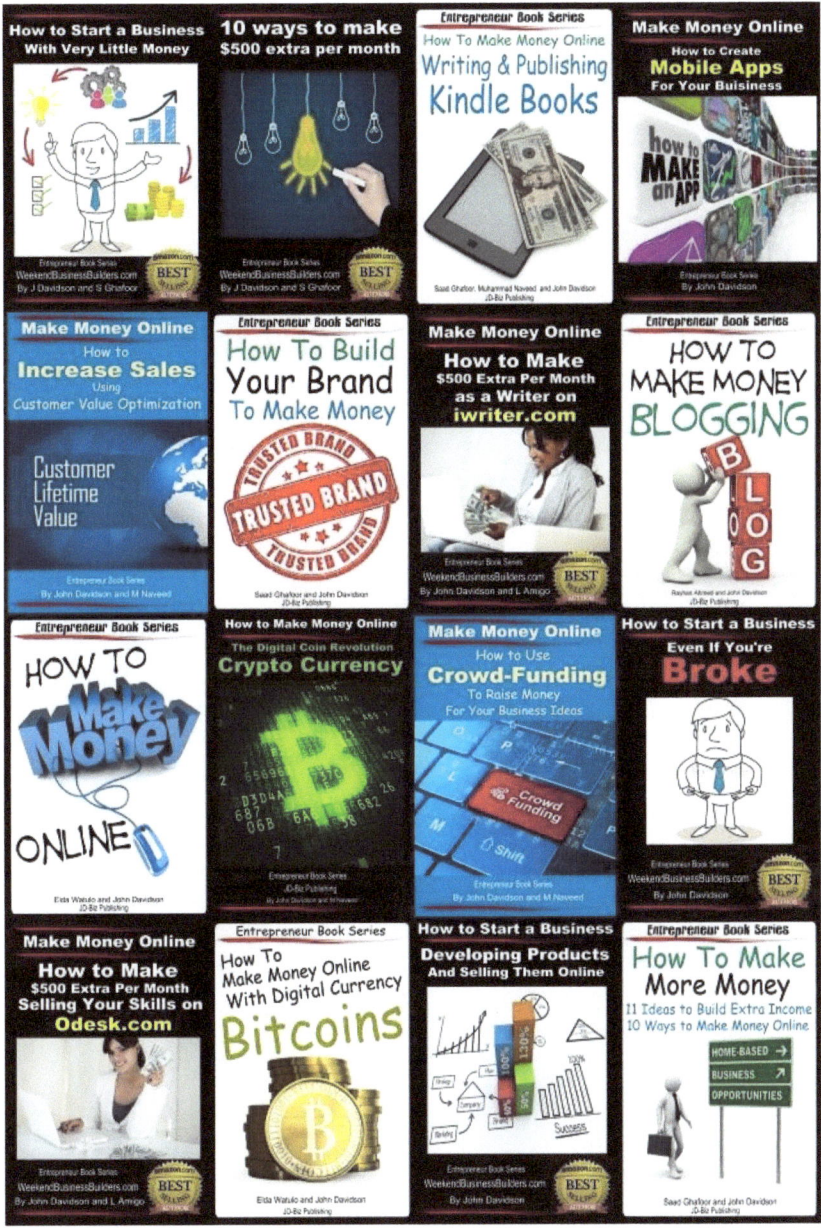

Our books are available at

1. Amazon.com
2. Barnes and Noble
3. Itunes
4. Kobo
5. Smashwords
6. Google Play Books

Download Free Books!

http://MendonCottageBooks.com

Publisher

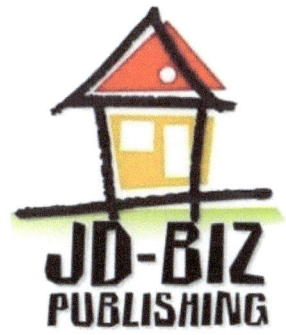

JD-Biz Corp

P O Box 374

Mendon, Utah 84325

http://www.jd-biz.com/

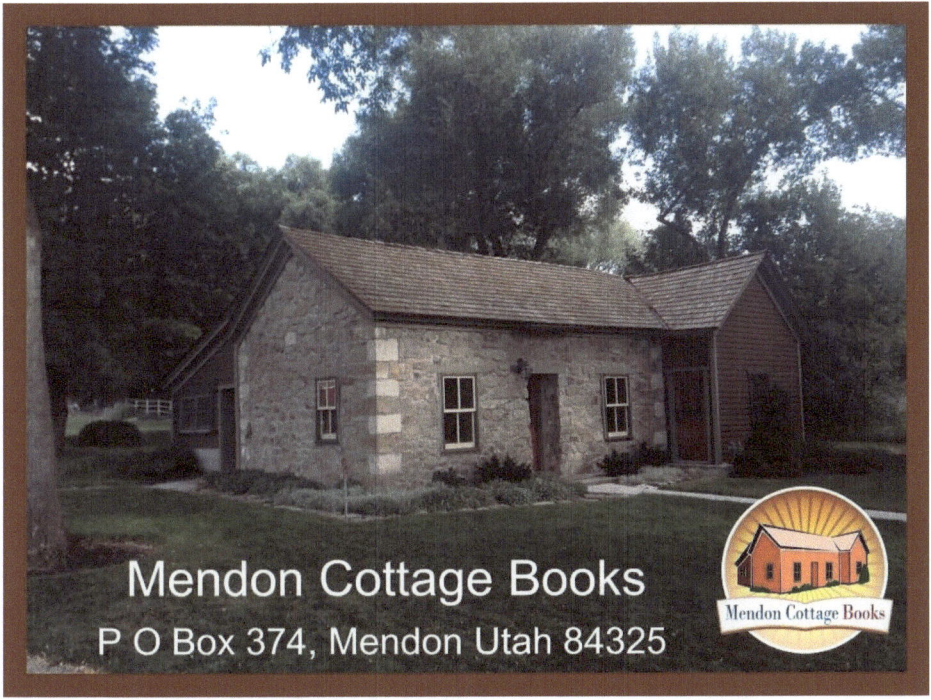